JUST SAY

# NO
TO
# DRUG
# TESTS

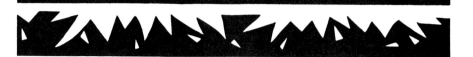

JUST SAY

# NO

TO

# DRUG TESTS

## HOW TO BEAT THE WHIZ QUIZ

ED CARSON

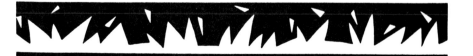

**PALADIN PRESS**
**BOULDER, COLORADO**

**Other titles by Ed Carson:**
B.A.D.: A Video Guide to Constructing and Firing Your Own
   Backyard Artillery Device

*Just Say No to Drug Tests:*
*How to Beat the Whiz Quiz*
by Ed Carson

Copyright © 1991 by Ed Carson

ISBN 10: 0-87364-624-X
ISBN 13: 978-0-87364-624-6
Printed in the United States of America

Published by Paladin Press, a division of
Paladin Enterprises, Inc.
Gunbarrel Tech Center
7077 Winchester Circle
Boulder, Colorado 80301 USA
+1.303.443.7250

Direct inquiries and/or orders to the above address.

Visit our Web site at www.paladin-press.com

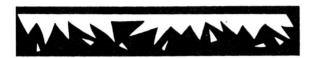

# CONTENTS

Introduction       1

*Chapter 1*
Testing Procedures       5

*Chapter 2*
Types of Tests       9

*Chapter 3*
Breathalyzers       13

*Chapter 4*
Drug Dogs       17

*Chapter 5*
Everyday Living       19

*Chapter 6*
Fooling the Test: Countermeasures       23

*Chapter 7*
Drug Testing and the Law       37

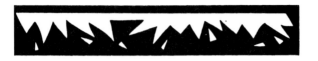

# WARNING

The use of drugs and the techniques described in this book can be dangerous. This book is not a legal or medical manual. Neither the author nor the publisher assumes any responsibility or liability for the use or misuse of information contained herein. Persons seeking to avoid the consequences of a positive drug or alcohol test should consult an attorney regarding their legal rights and a physician regarding their medical condition. *This book is for information purposes only.*

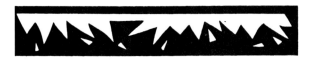

# INTRODUCTION

**THE FOURTH AMENDMENT** to the U.S. Constitution protects people's privacy and limits the government's power to search their homes and businesses:

*"The right of the people to be secure in their persons, houses, papers, and effects, against unreasonable searches and seizures, shall not be violated, and no warrants shall issue, but upon probable cause, supported by oath or affirmation, and particularly describing the place to be searched, and the persons or things to be seized."*

In 1791, when the Bill of Rights was ratified, it was not possible to search an individual's body fluids. Otherwise, I'm sure "body fluids" would have been included in the Fourth Amendment. The U.S. Supreme Court, however, is of the opinion that our founding fathers would have found urinalysis testing acceptable in any form.

There are many horror stories of people losing jobs, pensions, and benefits because of false-positive urinalysis test results. Most drug tests are not 100 percent accurate, and furthermore, many drug testing labs do not follow procedures necessary to obtain accurate results. This means false-positive and false-negative test results are realities, not just remote possibilities.

At least half of the Fortune 500 companies required pre-employment urinalysis testing in 1990. Members of the U.S. armed forces and federal civilian employees are also subject not only to pre-employment testing, but to probable-cause and random drug testing as well. The constitutional rights of these people and anyone else subject to urinalysis testing are being violated. With regard to the current ultraconservative Supreme Court, urinalysis drug testing is likely to be with us for awhile.

I have personally taken more than 150 urinalysis tests, and while I came up "dirty" on the first one, I have passed every test since. The tests I submitted to were administered by the U.S. government and a county probation program. This book details the techniques I used for eight years to fool the labs that were testing my urine.

The first part of this book is dedicated to explaining how urine samples are gathered, shipped, and tested. It is important to understand the different tests in order to defeat them effectively. This is followed by information on the different types of drug tests, including Breathalyzers that test for alcohol. There is also a chapter pertaining to the subject of drug dogs, because while it doesn't fall under drug testing per se, it is closely related to the issue of drugs and unconstitutional search and seizure.

Chapter 5 provides general tips for everyday avoidance of drug use detection, and Chapter 6 offers more detailed information on the techniques that can be used effectively to cleanse the body of drugs in order to pass a drug test. It then lists the various classes of drugs (including steroids), describes the use and action of each, and, according to the amount of time between when a particular drug was last taken and when a test is to be given, outlines specific day-by-day instructions for ridding the body of that drug in order to avoid detection. Also included in Chapter 6 is pertinent information about drugs and other substances that can be used to throw a test off, as well as ways to legitimize the presence of a particular class of drugs in your urine. Finally, the use of substitute urine samples as a last resort is discussed.

Chapter 7 is a brief overview of the laws relating to drug testing. For detailed information on the laws pertaining to drug testing, it is strongly suggested that you consult an attorney.

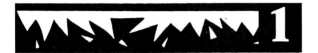

# TESTING
# PROCEDURES

**WHETHER YOU HAVE TO** take a pre-employment, random, or probable-cause urinalysis test, the urine is collected in the same way. Procedures vary slightly between different facilities but, overall, tight security measures are maintained in order for the test results to be considered valid. As soon as the sample is provided, a chain of custody is established—that is, each person who handles the sample thereafter must sign a form that stays with that sample and is kept with the test results at the lab. That form should have five blank lines and be signed by at least five different people, including the test administrator, the courier, the person who receives the sample at the lab, the lab technician, and the person who places the remainder of the sample in storage in case the results are disputed at a later date. If you notice a missing link in the chain of custody on a positive test result (e.g., a missing signature, two signatures by the same person, etc.) or the form is simply missing, contact an attorney.

The following are the security measures—and the intended purpose of each—used by one of the biggest drug testing laboratories in the country. Individuals being tested are required to:

1) *Sign the urinalysis consent form.* This is for the paranoid who will confess drug use and save the cost of the test.

2) *Show their driver's license.* This is to prevent people from having a relative or friend take the test for them.

3) *Put their name and Social Security number on the chain of custody form.* This establishes the chain of custody.

4) *List all prescription and nonprescription drugs used in the last month.* Various drugs will alter the results of a urinalysis test. These are discussed in Chapter 6.

5) *Remove their coats, roll up their shirt sleeves to expose their forearms, and push down their socks to expose their calves.* This prevents people from hiding someone else's urine on their person and presenting it as their own for testing.

6) *Remove all items from their shirt and pants pockets; no purses are allowed into the bathroom.*

7) *Wash their hands with soap and water, then towel dry.* This washes away salt or other foreign substances from being hidden under the fingernails and put in the sample bottle, which would produce a false-negative test result.

8) *Take the plastic seal off the specimen bottle issued to them and fill it at least halfway with urine.* The seal ensures that the bottle hasn't been tampered with.

9) *Be monitored until they provide a sample.* Like number 5, this prevents people from crotching someone else's urine and presenting it as their own.

10) *Take a lid and a tape seal from the test administrator, put the lid on tight, and place the tape seal across the lid and the side of the specimen bottle.* This is for chain of custody.

Once all of these steps have been completed, the attendant is instructed to take the bottle from the person and make sure that the sample is warm, as fresh urine in a bottle will feel quite warm to the touch.

As you can see, security is set up to be tight. Many facilities also add a dark blue dye to the toilet water to prevent people from adding water from the toilet to the sample in order to dilute it. (Dark blue urine would look quite strange.)

If you are going to be tested on an ongoing basis, note any ways in which your first test differs from the above procedure, then respond accordingly on your next test.

Chapter 6 includes a discussion on foreign substances that may be slipped into a sample to affect the results. In general, if you are going to bring something into the test to be used in this way, crotch it. Women have an easier time slipping some foreign substance into the sample because women's rest rooms have stall doors, whereas men are required to use urinals.

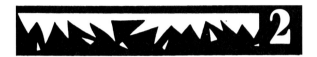

# TYPES OF TESTS

THERE ARE SEVERAL TYPES of tests used to detect drugs in urine. Most are capable of detecting several drugs during the same test, but some are more accurate than others. There are strict controls that labs follow to obtain the most accurate test results possible.

Test results are measured in nanograms per milliliter. That means one milliliter is broken into one billion parts. If seventy-five parts of that one billion is identified as cocaine, for example, you're busted! The cutoff between positive and negative might be fifty; forty-nine is negative and fifty is positive. Results are expressed as "parts per billion," or PPB.

As you see, the tests are very sensitive and precise. Think about it. One milliliter is about the size of a glass of water, which test procedures break into one billion pieces. This is precision.

There are several field tests available in which a tester simply puts a drop of urine on a chemically treated sheet of paper; if the paper changes color, drugs are detected.

Thin-layer chromatography (TLC) is capable of detecting about forty different drugs at one time. This test is done by mixing a drop of urine with a gel-like substance and spreading the mixture over a microscope slide. One edge of the slide is then dipped into a chemical solvent, which is pulled across the slide by the gel. The solvent and the gel separate the different chemicals found in the urine and organize them into different groups. Each group is left on a different location on the slide. Each spot that appears on the slide indicates the presence of a different drug. Lab technicians can tell by the size and color of each spot how much of a drug is present. If there are no drugs in a urine sample, no spots are left on the slide. Costing between ten and twenty-five dollars per test, TLC is one of the cheapest procedures available. It is generally used only as a screening test. If the results from this test come up positive, the urine is sent on for a confirmation test.

Enzyme immunoassy (EIA) is only able to test for ten drugs at a time. This test uses a machine that has ten different channels, each of which tests for a different drug. A drop of urine is put into each separate channel, and the machine adds two different chemicals or enzymes to each channel. The first chemical is designed to react with a certain drug, and if it does so, the second chemical changes color. If no drugs are present, the first chemical doesn't react, and no color change takes place. After the chemicals are mixed, the samples are passed in front of a light and photographed. All ten channels are photographed at once. A technician can tell by the intensity of the color how much of each channel's drug is present. A photograph will be white when no drugs are present. Costing between twenty-five and thirty-five dollars, the EIA test was the first to be used commercially and is still one of the most popular screening tests used today. The results from an

EIA test are usually used only for screening.

Radioimmunoassy (RIA) is much like the EIA test, using a machine that has ten channels, but RIA uses radiation rather than enzymes to detect drugs. Again, a drop of urine is put into each channel, and the machine adds a chemical, which is the same as the first chemical used in the EIA test. The second chemical is radioactive and sticks to the drug molecule. Each channel is then measured for radioactivity. If a channel shows no radioactivity, that channel's drug isn't present. RIA costs between twenty-five and thirty-five dollars per test; however, the machine is much more expensive than the EIA machine, and RIA technicians require more training. RIA is generally used only as a screening test.

Gas chromatography/mass spectrometry (GC/MS) can test for any known drug or chemical. It uses a huge machine that may cost more than twenty thousand dollars. In the GC/MS test, a drop of urine is put into a tube at one end of the machine. The urine is then vaporized and turned into a gas. A chemical is added that separates the urine into molecules. The computer then analyzes and identifies each molecule and prints out exactly what drugs and chemicals were in the urine in what quantity. If no drugs are present, the machine will show the salts and minerals present in all urine. Each test run costs between fifty and eighty dollars, and technicians receive extensive training before using the GC/MS machine. The GC/MS test is the only one that has proven to be 100 percent accurate.

Because of the costs involved in drug testing, most companies use the less accurate TLC, EIA, or RIA as screening tests. When a sample comes up positive, a GC/MS is then run as a confirmation test. This brings the total costs of a positive test to about $120.

What these tests can't tell is when a drug was taken and whether it was used or abused. Your employer doesn't own you twenty-four hours a day, and if your drug usage doesn't affect your job, it is none of your employer's business.

# 3

# BREATHALYZERS

BREATHALYZERS ARE MUCH more difficult to fool than any other substance testing device. Drug tests indicate drug use but can't tell how much or when. A breathalyzer can tell with great accuracy how much alcohol was used and whether a person is actually under the influence at the time of the test.

Alcohol is absorbed into your bloodstream through your stomach and intestines. When you breathe, your lungs exchange carbon dioxide in your blood for oxygen. Some of the alcohol in your blood is given off when you exhale, and this is what a breathalyzer measures. The results are given as your blood alcohol content (BAC).

There are more than thirty different breathalyzers on the market today, most of which use a technology called infrared absorption. A beam of infrared light is passed through a tube in the breathalyzer containing the air that was breathed into the machine. At the end of the beam of light is a sensor that detects how much of the original light was absorbed by your breath. From this the microprocessor in the breathalyzer can calculate the amount of alcohol in your bloodstream.

There are three basic types of breathalyzers: active desktop, active hand-held, and passive. Not all models use infrared absorption. Some hand-held and passive models use a technology called hydrocarbon sensing. These models heat and burn the air passing across the sensor, then measure the electrical resistance of the residue.

Active hand-held breathalyzers are carried by police in squad cars. Check with an attorney to find out the state laws regarding hand-held models. Police generally use these only to assist them in determining the extent of alcohol impairment and whether or not an evidentiary test should be given at the police station. Most hand-held models do not have flow sensors and, therefore, will not alert the police if you are not blowing.

Passive alcohol sensors are the most dangerous because most people don't know they exist, yet almost every police flashlight has one built in. Have the police ever pulled you over and shined a flashlight in your face? If this has happened, you probably were subjected to a passive alcohol test and didn't even know it.

The best way to fool the passive sensor is to roll down your car windows as soon as you see the flashing lights behind you. Don't be obvious; do it inconspicuously in order to get any alcohol fumes out of the car. Most people blinded by a flashlight will yell directly into it, giving the police the best possible reading. Though the police have a good strategy, you can counter with a better one. Simply relax and hold your breath while the light is in your face. The cop will not get a reading and, with any luck, will go on to harass someone else. However, flunking one of these tests will give the officer probable cause to take you to the station and give you an evidentiary breathalyzer test.

The active desktop breathalyzer uses infrared absorption technology and has flow detectors that measure the amount of air being blown into the machine. This ensures that air from deep in the lungs is trapped by the machine in order to give the highest BAC reading.

The key to fooling the evidentiary breathalyzer is time. Your body will metabolize or process one ounce of alcohol per hour. If, for example, you slam six shots of tequila, your BAC will go up for the first hour and then go down each succeeding hour. In this situation, you have almost no chance of fooling the breathalyzer unless you stall and don't take the test for at least three hours (or you happen to weigh four hundred pounds).

If you drink six shots of tequila and are pulled over two hours later, stall. Explain that you want to talk to your attorney before you take the test. Then claim that his or her number is busy, for example. Go to the bathroom. Take a drink of water and swish it around in your mouth to remove any alcohol residue. Then actually try to contact your attorney for advice. If you don't have an attorney, pick one out of the phone book and do as he or she advises.

If you can't stall and the police demand that you take the test or they will record your refusal to take the test, you must make a decision. Do you still feel drunk? If you do and you have been unable to contact an attorney, you have the right to refuse the test. If you don't feel drunk and you haven't reached an attorney, it is probably best to take the test.

You might be familiar with the logic that it is better to refuse the test than to be convicted of drunk driving. In most states, the penalty for refusing the test involves the suspension of driving privileges (i.e., the driver's license).

Depending on the state, a DUI *conviction* accumulates "points" on the driver's license and becomes a black mark on your record for a number of years. Also, it may or may not involve suspension of driving privileges, among other things. If you are definitely drunk, then, and you refuse the test, you have a chance of avoiding a DUI conviction. This may or may not be advantageous in terms of insurance coverage. Also, the recent Supreme Court decision to allow videotapes of drunk drivers to be used as evidence in court should be considered if you intend to refuse a breathalyzer test.

Obviously, it is becoming nearly impossible to avoid being convicted if you are stopped for DUI and you are under the influence of alcohol. The best defense you have against the breathalyzer is probably to stall as long as possible. A friend of mine once stalled for two hours before taking the test and blew a .07, which would have been at least a 1.0 if he hadn't stalled.

Under no circumstances should you agree to take a blood test. The BAC is always higher with a blood test when compared to a breathalyzer taken at the same time.

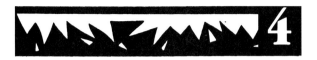

# DRUG DOGS

I ONCE SAW A DRUG DOG PICK out a car with a roach in the ashtray from a distance of twenty-five feet. I also saw a drug dog pass by a person who had an ounce of marijuana without detecting it. This was in Miami International Airport, and the dog was a U.S. Customs drug dog.

There is no doubt that the nose of a drug dog is extremely sensitive. Dogs that are specially trained to do so can sniff out all kinds of things, including explosives, cocaine (in the form of coke, freebase, or crack), and marijuana (in the form of hashish, hash oil, Thai-stick, THC capsules, and even resin). Be aware that marijuana pipes (bowls and bongs) are the easiest things for a drug dog to find. The resin that builds up in a pipe reeks and cannot be hidden from a drug dog. Do not take a pipe into an area that a drug dog might search—it will be found, and since resin is technically a form of marijuana, you may be charged with possession.

On the other hand, marijuana and cocaine may be hidden from a drug dog if an airtight barrier is created to prevent the dog from tracking the scent to its source. This must be done very carefully.

Put the drug into a plastic baggie. Wash your hands. Squeeze all of the air out of the baggie and seal the open end with a lighter. Wash your hands. Put that baggie into another baggie and seal it with a lighter. Wash your hands. Repeat this at least two more times. Use new baggies and wash your hands with soap and water to remove any drug residue.

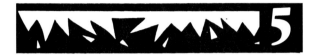

# EVERYDAY LIVING

YOUR BODY CHEMISTRY IS VERY complicated. Small changes in what you eat, drink, and do greatly affect how quickly your body cleans waste from its cells. Cell waste contains drug residue that ends up in your urine and is detected by drug tests. It is important to get rid of as much of this residue as possible before taking a urinalysis test. Don't wait until the day of the test to try to get rid of drug residue.

Blood delivers oxygen and nutrients to every cell in your body. It also collects waste from each cell, including drug residue. Your blood is then filtered by your kidneys, and all cell waste is removed. Your kidneys then deliver impurities to your bladder, where they are stored until you urinate.

Most drug residue is stored in fat cells throughout the body. (Steroids used by athletes are the exception, as they remain in muscle fiber.) The more body fat you have, the more drug residue you will carry around. A person who smokes one joint every day and is fifty pounds overweight is much less likely to pass a drug test than a fit person who smokes the same amount.

Check with a physician to find out what your percentage of body fat is. If it falls within a range that is considered "ideal," your chances of passing a drug test are significantly improved. If you are male, 15 to 20 percent body fat or less is considered ideal; if you are female, this increases to 20 to 25 percent or less. If you discover that your body fat percentage is above these levels, you are advised to use a physician-approved weight-loss and exercise program to reduce it.

Fluid intake is also important for flushing drugs from your body. The more fluids you pass through your body, the more drug residue you will flush out. Some fluids are better than others at cleansing. Cranberry juice is the best, but any fruit juice will work. Alcohol and beer are terrible and, in fact, are counterproductive because they place such a load on your kidneys that less drug residue is filtered out.

Maintain a high fluid intake at all times. Get into the habit of drinking an additional one-half gallon of fluids per day than normal. If you know you will be tested in one week, for instance, increase that to one gallon over and above what you would normally drink on a daily basis. This is especially important if you are tested at random.

Another thing you want to watch is salt intake. Salt often causes your body to retain fluids, which is exactly what you don't want. You want the fluids to flow in and right back out so that your body continues to cleanse itself.

Probable-cause tests are routinely administered by the military and some private employers (those in public transportation, for example) whenever someone is involved in an accident on the job. This is about the only type of test you can avoid. If you don't take chances or risks that might get you in trouble and you don't give your employer probable cause to suspect that you are using drugs, you are less likely to be tested.

A few final thoughts here. Don't overuse. If you are already stoned, don't spark up another. Avoid peer pressure. And remember: friends come and go, but enemies last forever. In other words, don't make enemies and set yourself up for blackmail, which could get you tested.

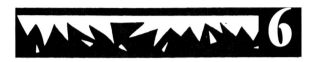

# FOOLING THE TEST: COUNTERMEASURES

LET'S BEGIN BY REVIEWING the techniques that can be used to cleanse the body of the various drugs. In the second part of this chapter, you will find the various categories of drugs listed, along with brief descriptions of their use and action as well as ways of legitimizing or masking their presence in your urine. You will then be given a set of specific instructions to follow, depending upon how much time you have before the test.

## CLEANSING TECHNIQUES

### Kidney Shape-Up

Kidney shape-up is necessary so that your kidneys filter as much drug residue from your blood as possible. The more drug residue you remove from your body in the weeks prior to the test, the less likely it is that your test will come up positive for a particular drug.

To do this, you must not consume any alcohol—and this includes beer—in the time prior to testing. Avoid fatty foods, including fried foods, red meat, and butter, among others, and eat lots of vegetables. The most important thing you should do is drink a lot of cranberry juice—at least two liters a day is recommended.

*Water Dilution*

Water dilution is one of the most important techniques. The more fluids that pass through your body, the more drug residue you remove. You must greatly increase your water intake before the test. This also involves drinking as many fluids as possible on the day of the test, because at that point, you may still have a certain amount of drug residue in your body.

The more fluids you mix with the remaining residue, the more diluted that residue will be. Remember, the drug residue in your body must exceed a certain level in order to flunk a test. Just because three molecules of THC are found does not mean you will flunk.

Drink at least two gallons of fluids—fruit juices or water—every day before the test. (Again, no alcohol, and avoid salt, which causes water retention.) Also take vitamin C tablets (500-1,000 mg. per day) during this time; the acid in vitamin C helps remove the drug residue from fatty tissue. Another cleanser is golden seal root, available at most health food stores. Be sure to get the root and not just the herb, which is not as effective. Take at least one tablet or capsule every day before the test.

Spending as much time as possible in a sauna is also very important. Drink a lot of cranberry juice before going into the sauna. When you sweat you lose body fluids as well as drug residue; in addition to having cleansing properties, cranberry juice will help replace these fluids. Take a sauna at least three times per week. Stay in as long as you can stand it, take a ten-minute break, and repeat.

Another important part of water dilution is fasting. Fast at least one day per week. Fasting consists of eating no breakfast or lunch and having only a salad for dinner. For dressing, use a little bit of Italian or vinaigrette, or better yet, just vinegar, which is available in flavored varieties. The acids in vinegar are helpful for breaking down fat. Fasting for short periods will help you burn up fatty tissue that contains drug residue. Do not fast on the day of the test.

### Exercise

Develop an intensive aerobic exercise program to help burn fatty tissue and cleanse the body of drug residue through perspiration. You should exercise for at least thirty minutes per day. Break a sweat—don't just go through the motions.

### Kidney Shutdown

You should drink a lot of fluids in general on the day of the test and try to urinate frequently. This will flush as much remaining drug residue as possible from your body. Then you must shut your kidneys down so that any residue that might be left in the cells will not be filtered into the urine. This is accomplished by drinking vinegar about two to three hours before the test. Take 2 fluid ounces per 50 pounds of body weight. For example, if you weigh 150 pounds, you should drink 6 ounces of vinegar. (A shot glass holds 1 fluid ounce.) When you drink the vinegar, be sure to burp between each shot. If you fail to do so, you are likely to vomit. Some people prefer apple cider vinegar over regular vinegar. Some people find it easier to mix the vinegar with a glass of juice. I prefer straight white vinegar chased by a glass of orange juice.

## DRUGS

Now that you have a thorough understanding of the methods for cleansing the body of drugs, simply look up the drug that concerns you, estimate the time between when that drug was last taken and the testing date, and follow the procedure indicated.

### Amphetamines

Today, true prescription amphetamines are hard to come by on the street, but the sale and use of crystal meth and ice (pure methamphetamine powder produced illegally in labs) are reportedly on the rise. There are also many types of fake speed on the street that actually contain only a mixture of caffeine and phenylpropanolamine (PPA). This is the same combination that is found in many diet pills. This so-called "speed" comes in the shape and color of prescription amphetamines–"black beauties," "Christmas trees," "brown and clears," "speckled eggs," "pink hearts," and "footballs." Most of the fakes will sell for about fifty cents a hit on the street, while prescription speed sells for about five dollars a hit. It is perfectly legal to manufacture and sell the fakes because they do not contain amphetamine (although the Food and Drug Administration is considering ways to crack down on this). It is also legal to use these. However, professional and amateur athletes are often tested for abnormal levels of caffeine.

A prescription for an amphetamine will invalidate any urine test that comes up positive for amphetamines. If you can get a prescription from a doctor, take it with you to the test. For some time, amphetamines were widely accepted as a weight-loss method. Some physicians will still prescribe amphetamines for weight problems, although they are becoming increasingly cautious about doing so because of problems with addiction and the proliferation of eating disorders such as anorexia. There are no other drugs that will throw off the test.

If it is not possible to obtain a prescription for amphetamines, the following procedures are recommended:

*One to two months before the test:* stop using, kidney shape-up, water dilution, kidney shutdown on the day of the test (optional).

*Less than one month before the test:* stop using, kidney shape-up, water dilution, kidney shutdown on the day of the test.

### Barbiturates

Barbiturates include phenobarbital, amobarbital, and secobarbital or Seconal. Barbiturates are made from malonic acid, found in apples and also urea, which is part of human urine. This makes it difficult to detect barbiturates through urinalysis. In addition, almost any trace of barbiturates disappears from the body naturally within seven days of their last use.

It is becoming increasingly difficult to get a prescription for barbiturates. In the past, they were widely prescribed for a variety of physical and psychological problems. But again, because of problems with addiction, physicians have become increasingly wary of this. Also, new drugs that are capable of treating various mild psychoses more specifically than barbiturates have become available in recent years. Barbiturates are still used for some things, such as controlling seizures, however. If you are able to get a prescription, of course, positive test results cannot be held against you because you obtained the drug legally under the direction of a physician.

*One to two weeks before the test:* stop using, kidney shape-up, water dilution, kidney shutdown on the day of the test (optional).

*Less than one week before the test:* stop using, water dilution, kidney shutdown on the day of the test.

### Cocaine

Once again, crack and freebase are included in this category. On the average, all traces of cocaine disappear from the urine within five days of its last use. Some people are clean in three days, and for others it may take as long as a week. This happens naturally, without any actions needed to speed the process. There is no way to obtain a prescription for cocaine to legitimize its presence in your urine, and there are no other drugs that will fool the test.

*One to two weeks before the test:* stop using, kidney shape-up, water dilution, kidney shutdown on the day of the test (optional).

*One day to one week before the test:* stop using, kidney shape-up, water dilution, kidney shutdown on the day of the test.

### Diazepam

Included in this category are Librium and Valium, both of which are sedatives. Diazepam can be detected in urine up to one month after its last use.

It is relatively easy to get a prescription for Valium (it is one of the most widely prescribed drugs in the United States), which would legitimize test results that come up positive for diazepam. Complaining of nervousness, anxiety, or sleeplessness will generally get you a prescription for Valium. There are no drugs that will mask the use of diazepam.

*Four to six weeks before the test:* stop using, kidney shape-up, water dilution, kidney shutdown on the day of the test (optional).

*Less than one month before the test:* stop using, kidney shape-up, water dilution, kidney shutdown on the day of the test.

### Hallucinogens

Lysergic acid diethylamide (LSD), mescaline (peyote buttons), and psilocybin (mushrooms) are hallucinogens. They each have different active chemicals, but none are detectable by blood or urine tests. The reason for this is that the amount of each drug that a person would take to get high is minute. For example, there are only four nanograms of lysergic acid in an average hit of blotter acid (a type of LSD). The minimum standards used by drug testing labs vary, but they are hundreds of times higher than this. To my knowledge, there are no labs that look for hallucinogens.

### Opiates

Opiates include codeine, opium, heroin, morphine, Demerol (meperidine), and sometimes Thai-stick (often soaked in opium oil), all of which are detectable by urinalysis. Most labs will test for opiates.

If you have used opiates, you should go to a doctor and complain of a bad cough that's keeping you awake at night and try to get a prescription for a cough syrup that contains codeine. Another possibility is to try to get a prescription for Tylenol 3, which also contains codeine and is often prescribed for low-level pain. If you provide your prescription when tested, any opiate that shows up on the test can't be held against you because you have proof that you took codeine prescribed by a physician. While urinalysis can detect the presence of an opiate, it is unable to differentiate between heroin and Tylenol 3.

If you are unable to get a prescription, the following procedures are recommended to cleanse your body of opiates.

*Three to five weeks before the test:* stop using, kidney shape-up, water dilution, fasting, kidney shutdown on the day of the test (optional).

*One to three weeks before the test:* stop using, kidney shape-up, water dilution, fasting, kidney shutdown on the day of the test.

*Less than one week before the test:* stop using, kidney shape-up, water dilution, fasting, kidney shutdown on the day of the test.

If you have less than one week, you will have to double the recommended water intake and spend more time in the sauna. With less than three days before a test, you will have to use substitute urine (refer to the end of this chapter).

### Phencyclidine (PCP)

PCP is one of the most difficult drugs to clean from your body. It can appear in urine tests up to six months after just one use. It goes without saying, then, that PCP should be avoided at all costs in situations where drug testing is possible.

There is no way to obtain a prescription for PCP to legitimize its use, and there are no other drugs that will mess up the test.

*One to six months before the test:* stop using, kidney shape-up, water dilution, intense exercise, kidney shutdown on the day of the test.

*Less than one month before the test:* stop using, kidney shape-up, water dilution, intense exercise, kidney shutdown on the day of the test.

### Quaaludes

Methaqualone (Quaalude) is detectable by urinalysis, but I am not aware of any labs that look for the presence of methaqualone in urine. The reason for this is that methaqualone has not been made legally since 1980. There were some bootleg 'ludes going around until 1982, but these were not real Quaaludes. They contained no methaqualone and usually were made from diazepam (the active chemical in Valium). I have not seen or heard of any bootleg quaaludes since 1982, but if you have, refer to the section on diazepam.

### Tetrahydrocannabinol (THC)

The presence of THC, which can come from marijuana, hashish, and Thai-stick, can be detected by urinalysis up to six months after chronic use by an overweight person. On the other hand, I know of one case in which a person who was in good shape passed a test just one day after smoking a joint.

The chemical makeup of THC is such that it is broken down very slowly by the body. However, because it is stored in fat cells, one of the most important tricks to passing a test for THC is reducing your percentage of body fat. If you are male, you should have 15 to 20 percent body fat or less. If you are female, 20 to 25 percent body fat or less is the range you want to strive for. (Refer to

Chapter 5 for more information on this.)

Prescriptions for THC are rare; it is generally prescribed only to relieve the side effects of chemotherapy. But one thing you can do is include pain relievers containing ibuprofen on the list of prescription and nonprescription drugs that you will file with the testing facility. If you actually take four on the morning of the test, this will confuse EIA and RIA test machines. (The explanation is long and complicated, but it does work.) If you can get away with it, adding some table salt to your urine sample will also help throw off the test results, especially with EIA and RIA tests. The fast-food packs of salt are ideal for this; only use about half of the salt in the packet.

In addition, the following procedures will help cleanse your body of THC:

*Two to four weeks (or more) before the test:* stop using, kidney shape-up, water dilution, kidney shutdown on the day of the test (optional).

*Less than two weeks before the test:* stop using, kidney shape-up, water dilution, kidney shutdown on the day of the test.

Again, percentage of body fat is the key to passing a THC urine test.

## ATHLETIC PERFORMANCE ENHANCERS

Almost any athlete competing above the high school level is subject to drug testing. There are almost as many drugs used by athletes as there are sports. Some athletic performance enhancers are not drugs at all. Some performance-enhancing techniques use human hormones (or synthetic derivatives thereof), and others use the athlete's own blood. Some of these techniques are presently undetectable by urine or blood samples.

Because of the publicity and large amounts of money spent on athletics, drug testing labs are spending increasingly greater amounts of time and money on developing accurate, foolproof athletic drug tests and less time on recreational drug tests. (In fact, recreational drug testing technology has changed little in the last ten years.)

### Blood Doping

Currently, blood doping is not detectable by blood test or urinalysis. Only a blood test could detect this technique, and it appears as if it will be ten years or more before such a test is developed. Athletes who use blood doping remove one or two pints of blood six to eight weeks before the competition. The blood is separated, and only the red blood cells are kept. During this six- to eight-week period, an athlete's body replaces the blood that was removed. Then, before the competition, the red blood cells are injected back into the athlete. This excess of red blood cells enables more oxygen to be carried to the muscles during the event, increasing energy levels and enhancing endurance. It is, of course, inadvisable to use anyone else's blood, because of the risks involved with AIDS and hepatitis, among other things.

### Beta Blockers

Beta blockers calm the nerves. These have been used, for example, by biathletes, pool players, and archers. They are detectable by urinalysis, and there is no known way to hide or disguise them because they must be taken just prior to the competition.

### Anabolic Steroids

Anabolic steroids are the most widely used athletic

performance enhancers; they are also the most detectable by urinalysis. Anabolic steroids are usually used during training to build muscle mass. Included in this category are fluoxymesterone, nandrolone, norethandrolone, oxandrolone, stanozol, and testosterone. All of these are man-made, except testosterone, which occurs naturally in the human body. All except testosterone can be detected by the GC/MS test.

Because urine always contains testosterone, a test was developed that compares the level of epitestosterone, another hormone present in urine, to that of testosterone. If a person has a high level of testosterone in his or her urine compared to the level of epitestosterone, he or she is assumed to have taken testosterone illegally. Some athletes have begun taking epitestosterone along with testosterone in order to throw the test off. This renders the test ineffective since it is based on comparative levels of these hormones as opposed to actual levels. While the illegitimate use of testosterone is not presently detectable when used in conjunction with epitestosterone, it may be within the next five years.

All of the other anabolic steroids can be detected by urine tests, and they are difficult to disguise because they are stored in muscle tissue rather than fat cells. Steroids are commonly prescribed to athletes for sports-related injuries, but even if this were the case, their detection would generally disqualify an athlete from an event. Some athletes have used a drug called probenecid (used to treat gout) to mask steroid use. The steroids don't show up in the test results, but the probenecid does. Consequently, most professional and amateur sports commissions now test for probenecid.

The best way to avoid detection of anabolic steroids is to

stop using three to four weeks prior to the competition. However, most professional and amateur sports commissions are considering ways to implement testing during the training period prior to an event, which would make the use of these steroids almost obsolete. For the time being, if you must cleanse your body of one of these, this section should help.

*Four to six weeks before the test:* stop using, kidney shape-up, water dilution, intensive exercise.

*Less than one month before the test:* your only option is to use substitute urine (refer to the end of this chapter).

### Human Growth Hormone (HGH)

Human growth hormone (HGH) is undetectable because it is present in all people. At the base of the brain is a pea-sized gland called the pituitary, which produces HGH. Before and during puberty, production of HGH peaks. It then acts on other glands in the body and, in turn, these glands make testosterone and epitestosterone, along with about a dozen other hormones that make the body develop and grow.

Athletes take HGH in very small amounts compared to anabolic steroids. Many physicians feel that HGH is safer to use than anabolic steroids because it is not synthetic, and it uses the body's natural growth mechanisms by triggering the production of other hormones. (Anabolic steroids, in effect, skip the first step in the natural growth process. This is theorized to be the reason many athletes who use them eventually develop cancer.) However, this steroid is very expensive when compared with anabolic steroids because it can be obtained only from the human pituitary gland. It will probably be at least twenty years before there is a test capable of detecting the illegal use of HGH by athletes. Such a test would probably be based on genetic codes.

## SUBSTITUTE URINE SAMPLES

In some cases, people have successfully put another person's urine into their sample bottles and presented it for testing. This is risky for a number of reasons, but it is an option if you are subject to an unexpected test that you are sure you will flunk.

If this proves to be your only option, it is important to conceal the urine you sneak into the test near a warm part of your body. As mentioned earlier, most test lab procedures specify feeling the sample you provide to ensure that it is warm. It is also important to be certain that the person whose urine you substitute for your own is clean. It would be a shame to go to the trouble of sneaking urine into a test only to fail anyway.

As drug testing has proliferated, a number of companies have capitalized on the need for "clean urine." Some sell urine "certified" to be drug-free. Others sell freeze-dried urine–simply add water to the crystals and you have instant urine! Many of these companies advertise their product in weight lifting magazines, among other sources.

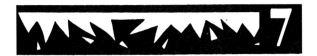

# DRUG TESTING
# AND THE LAW

WHERE LEGAL PROCEEDINGS ARE involved, the results of drug tests must be admissible as evidence in a court of law in order for them to be held against you. The admissibility in court of drug or alcohol test results depends upon the relevancy of those results and their probative value to the court proceedings. Not all drug test results are admissible against you for all purposes. This means that some results may not be used against you to prove intoxication or impairment, especially if the test that was used is not considered extremely accurate. However, most results will be admitted into evidence for some purpose. The rules of evidence vary depending on the jurisdiction.

To evaluate the accuracy of the various tests available, labs were provided with urine samples containing measured amounts of drugs. The results each machine showed were compared with the actual amounts of drugs known to be contained in the original samples.

The GC/MS was the only one shown to be accurate 100 percent of the time. Therefore, it is admissible as evidence in court as long as it can be demonstrated that the sample's chain of custody was maintained. It would be almost impossible to prove to a court that a GC/MS result was wrong.

The EIA and RIA tests have been shown to be inaccurate 5 to 10 percent of the time. It would be difficult to convict someone of drug use based on test results that can be wrong that often. This and the high cost of the GC/MS test are the reasons EIA and RIA are used as screening tests, while the GC/MS test is used for confirmation.

It is important that you note the difference between civil and criminal liability. Civil liability arises in lawsuits filed against you to recover damages (the person you greased while driving drunk sues to recover monetary damages for injuries incurred). Criminal liability arises when you violate federal, state, or local law that imposes criminal penalties (you get popped by a state trooper for driving drunk and go to jail). Generally, administrative penalties may be imposed separately and in addition to criminal penalties. If you refuse to take a breathalyzer, for instance, you may lose your driving privileges for a year (administrative penalty). That does not, however, preclude a criminal conviction for DUI based on testimony of the arresting officer and witnesses (your buddies at the local saloon) and other incriminating evidence (a videotape of your interrogation at the police station). Laws governing civil, criminal, and administrative liability vary, depending on the jurisdiction.

In a criminal prosecution, the defendant's commission of the crime must be proven beyond a reasonable doubt. In a civil case, the plaintiff usually must prove the case by a preponderance of evidence. In other words, the scale of evidence must be tipped in favor of the plaintiff.

If your job involves public transportation and there is

an accident, you could be forced to take a drug test because the accident is considered probable cause. If you flunk it, you could be charged criminally. If you apply for a job involving public transportation and you are asked to take a drug test and fail it, you probably will not be charged or convicted, but you won't get the job.

Obviously, the issue of drug testing and the law is a complicated one. When drug testing concerns you, it is always advisable to seek the advice of an attorney who can fill you in on local laws and your legal rights. Do not attempt to represent yourself in court on a drug-testing matter. As the saying goes, "One who is self-represented in court has a fool for a client."